The Fight Against Insomnia

A Nutritionist's Guide - Change Your Diet and Banish Insomnia for Good.

By Laura Hails

Contents

Introduction

Insomnia is a very common problem that takes a toll on your energy, mood, and ability to function during the day. Chronic insomnia can even contribute to serious health problems. It is estimated that as many as 30 percent of adults suffer from some form of insomnia and many turn to medication in an attempt to solve the problem.

But you don't have to resign yourself to sleepless nights. The good news is that most cases of insomnia can be cured with changes you can make on your own, just a few tweaks in your diet may be all that is needed to end insomnia for good. Common vitamins and minerals found in certain foods have been shown to improve both the quality and duration of sleep. By addressing the underlying causes and making simple changes to your sleep environment and your diet you can put a stop to the frustration of insomnia and finally get a good night's sleep.

The food we eat creates the person that we become, eat healthy, nutritious food and you will look radiant, have more energy, become more active, sleep more soundly, lose excess weight and ultimately, achieve more.

This book will explain what a nutritious diet should look like, tips on how to introduce a healthy diet into your life coupled with an explanation of the specific foods that you should be consuming more of to help you banish insomnia from your life for good and to finally reap the benefits of a regular good night's sleep.

Chapter One

Insomnia

What is Insomnia

Insomnia is the inability to fall asleep or stay asleep at night, resulting in unrefreshing or non-restorative sleep. Because different people need different amounts of sleep, insomnia is defined by the quality of your sleep and how you feel after sleeping—not the number of hours you sleep or how quickly you doze off. Even if you're spending eight hours a night in bed, if you feel drowsy and fatigued during the day, you may be experiencing insomnia.

Although insomnia is the most common sleep complaint, it is not a single sleep disorder. It's more accurate to think of insomnia as a symptom of another problem. The problem causing the insomnia differs from person to person. It could be something as simple as drinking too much caffeine during the day or a more complex issue like an underlying medical condition or feeling overloaded with responsibilities.

Symptoms of Insomnia –

Difficulty falling asleep despite being tired

Waking up frequently through the night

Trouble getting back to sleep when awakened in the night

Unrefreshed sleep

Relying on sleeping aids to get to sleep

Daytime drowsiness, fatigue or irritability

Difficulty concentrating through the day

Common causes of insomnia

Before changing our diet to combat insomnia it is important to find the root cause of your sleepless nights. Making small changes to your lifestyle combined with a diet that is not only nutritious but that also includes more of the right foods can illuminate insomnia and help you get your life back on track.

Whilst this book concentrates on changing your diet to fight insomnia, we should first look at the issues that might be causing your particular insomnia problems. Emotional issues such as stress, anxiety, and depression cause half of all insomnia cases. But your daytime habits, sleep routine, and physical health may also play a role. Try to identify all possible causes of your insomnia. Once you figure out the root cause, you can begin to experience the wonders of restful sleep.

- Are you under a lot of stress?

- Are you depressed?

- Do you struggle with feelings of anxiety?

- Have you recently gone through a traumatic experience?

- Are you taking any medications that might be affecting your sleep?

- Do you have any health problems that may be interfering with sleep?

- Is your sleep environment quiet and comfortable?

Reasons for Insomnia

Sometimes, insomnia only lasts a few days and goes away on its own, especially when the insomnia is tied to an obvious temporary cause. However, some people have it for years, many just come to terms with it as they have had it so long that they believe it is just something they have to put up with. Chronic insomnia is usually tied to an underlying mental or physical issue.

Anxiety, stress, and depression

Some of the most common causes of chronic insomnia are as a result of anxiety, stress and depression, issues that are all interlinked. Each of these symptoms can make the others worse. Understanding these underlying problems is an essential part of the road to recovery.

Medical problems or illness.

Many medical conditions and diseases can contribute to insomnia, including asthma, allergies, Parkinson's disease, hyperthyroidism, acid reflux, kidney disease, and cancer. Chronic pain is also a common cause of insomnia.

Medications.

Many prescription drugs can interfere with sleep, including antidepressants, stimulants for ADHD, corticosteroids, thyroid hormone, high blood pressure medications, and some contraceptives. Common over-the-counter culprits include cold and flu medications that contain alcohol, pain relievers that contain caffeine, diuretics, and slimming pills.

Breaking Bad Habits

Look at your daily habits, some of the things you're doing to cope with insomnia may actually be making the problem worse.

Are you using sleeping pills?

Are you drinking too much alcohol or caffeine before bedtime?

Are you drinking too much coffee through the day – caffeine can build up in your system and stay in it for up to 10 hours.

Do you have an irregular sleep pattern?

Do you nap through the day?

Do you eat too much sugar in the evening?

Do you eat heavy evening meals too close to bedtime?

Do you get enough exercise through the day?

Or too much exercise too close to bed time.

Identify poor daytime habits and break them where you can. Small changes can have big results.

Good Bedtime Habits to Introduce.

Ensure that you have a quiet, comfortable sleep environment and a relaxing bedtime routine.

Make sure your bedroom is quiet, dark, and cool.

Noise, light, and a bedroom that's too hot or cold, or an uncomfortable mattress or pillow can all interfere with sleep. Try using a sound machine or earplugs to mask outside noise, an open window or fan to keep the room cool, and blackout curtains or an eye mask to block out light. Ensure that you have the right mattress firmness and pillows that provide the support you need to sleep comfortably.

Stick to a regular sleep schedule.

Support your biological clock by going to bed and getting up at the same time every day, including weekends. Get up at your usual time in the morning even if you're tired. This will help you get back in a regular sleep rhythm.

Turn off all screens at least an hour before bed.

Electronic screens emit a blue light that disrupts your body's production of melatonin and combats sleepiness. So instead of watching TV or spending time on your phone, tablet, or computer, choose another relaxing activity, such as reading a book or listening to soft music.

Avoid stimulating activity and stressful situations before bedtime.

This includes checking messages on social media, big discussions or arguments with your spouse or family, or catching up on work. Postpone these things until the morning.

Avoid naps.

Napping during the day can make it more difficult to sleep at night. If you feel like you have to take a nap, limit it to 30 minutes before 3 p.m.

Drinking too many liquids.

Waking up at night to go to the bathroom becomes a bigger problem as we age. By not drinking anything an hour before sleep and going to the bathroom several times as you get ready for bed, you can reduce the frequency you'll wake up to go during the night.

Alcohol.

While a nightcap may help you to relax and fall asleep, it interferes with your sleep cycle once you fall asleep, causing broken sleep and quite often leaving you feeling unrefreshed in the morning.

Big evening meals.

Try to make dinnertime earlier in the evening, and avoid heavy, rich foods within two hours of bed. Spicy or acidic foods can cause stomach trouble and heartburn which can wake you during the night.

Caffeine.

Some studies suggest that if you suffer from insomnia you should avoid drinking caffeine at least six hours before bedtime. People who are sensitive to caffeine may need to stop even earlier.

Simple Changes

Simple changes to your evening habits like choosing protein foods that are rich in an amino acid called tryptophan. This helps boost the sleep-inducing hormone melatonin. Chicken and turkey, milk and dairy, nuts and seeds are all good choices.

Combine these with rice, pasta or potatoes to help the body get the most benefits from tryptophan. Try a chicken and noodle stir-fry or similar. Aim to eat your main meal earlier in the evening - the act of eating pushes up the body's core temperature and this can disrupt sleep so eat your evening meal at least 4 hours before retiring for the day.

Chapter Two
A Nutritional Diet

Proteins

Protein is a powerful nutrient, it plays a major role in our body, building body tissue and making important hormones. Proteins are made up of a collection of 20 amino acids, these are divided into two - "essential" which are sourced from your food and "non-essential that are produced by your body.

Protein, will keep you fuller for longer, it will help you concentrate, reduce sugar cravings, give you energy and keep your hair, nails and bones strong. The protein in your body is constantly being broken down and replaced. The body does not store amino acids like it does carbohydrates and fats, so it needs a daily supply of amino acids to make new proteins. The protein in the food you eat is digested into amino acids that can be used to replace the protein in your body.

There are two different types of proteins in our diet, complete and incomplete. The difference between the two is determined by its amino acid composition.

Complete Proteins – These are proteins that supply all "essential amino acids" complete proteins come from foods such as eggs, milk, meat, fish and soy.

Complete proteins are great sauces of protein and should make up 75% of our daily protein intake, however you can combine incomplete proteins with complete proteins to ensure you are getting the complete range of "essential amino acids" in your diet.

Animal Derived Complete Proteins – Meat, poultry, fish and shellfish all contain all the "essential" amino acids. Fish and shellfish are a particularly good source of complete protein because they are low fat and rich in essential minerals. Examples include shrimp, scallops, clams, tuna, salmon, mackerel, halibut, sardines and cod.

Vegetarian, Animal Derived Complete Proteins – Eggs and dairy products are also complete proteins, containing all essential amino acids. Examples are eggs, cheese and yoghurt. Quorn – although not derived from animals is a plant based complete protein but as it contains some dairy it cannot be classed as vegan.

Vegan, Plant Based Complete Proteins - Plant-based foods that are complete protein choices, include soy products, quinoa and buckwheat – which are a protein-rich whole grain. Soybeans form the basis of many processed soy foods, all of which are complete protein sources, such as soy milk, tempeh, tofu, miso and edamame which are fresh green soybeans.

Incomplete Proteins – These are proteins that do not contain all essential amino acids, or don't have sufficient quantities of them to meet the body's needs and should be combined with other proteins. Examples of incomplete proteins are nuts and seeds, pulses, grains such as rice and vegetables.

These proteins shouldn't be ignored as they contribute towards a healthy, balanced diet. Proteins that in combination with each other provide the complete range of essential amino acids are called complementary proteins. Complimentary proteins don't have to be combined at the same meal, but they should be combined within the same day as the body does not store the protein it consumes.

Examples of complementary proteins are – rice and beans, spinach and almonds, hummus and whole grain pittas.

Carbohydrates –

Dietary carbohydrates are split into three categories:

Sugars – these are short chain carbohydrates that are found in foods, examples of sugar carbohydrates are glucose,

Starches – these are long chains of glucose molecules, which eventually get broken down into glucose in the digestive system these are found in potatoes, corn and oats, peas and rice.

Fibre – Humans cannot digest fibre, but the bacteria in the digestive system can make use of some of them, fibre is essential for a healthy digestive system. Fibre is found in vegetables, fruit, salad, pulses and whole grains.

The most important thing to know about carbohydrates is that you need them to give you energy, by eating the right foods you naturally become more energetic, you do more, and you burn off more calories. A balanced diet helps with weight control, sleeping patterns and memory and concentration levels. The key is to eat the right carbs and ditch the wrong ones

Carbohydrates in their natural form are good for you and should be part of a healthy, balanced diet. Whilst cutting down on simple carbohydrates such as biscuits, cakes and pastries will increase your wellbeing and help you maintain a healthy diet you shouldn't be tempted to cut complex carbohydrates from your diet.

Carbohydrates are not essential as the body can function without them, however, complex carbohydrates are an important part of a healthy diet because of their high nutritional value. Cut back on simple carbohydrates and increase the complex ones.

The More Complex the better

Complex Carbs are starch and fibre and have more nutrients then Simple Carbs. They have a higher fibre content and therefore, digest more slowly making you feel fuller for longer.

Complex carbohydrates are more filling and therefore will help you control your weight, they also help keep your blood sugars level, which stops cravings.

Complex Carbohydrates you should be eating –

fruit, vegetables, nuts, pulses and whole grains, whole wheat bread and cereal, corn, oats, peas and brown or wild rice.

1 - whole grains – these are good sources of fibre, as well as potassium, magnesium and selenium. Choose - quinoa, buckwheat, and whole – wheat pasta and noodles

2 - Fruit – such as apples, berries and bananas.

3 - Vegetables – all vegetables, but in particular, leafy greens such as spinach, kale and cabbage.

4 - Beans – beans, peas and lentils.

<u>Fats –</u>

Good fats – Oil rich, nutritious foods like <u>nuts, seeds and avocados</u> are rich in omega 3 and 6 fatty acids which protect against heart disease, aid weight loss, lower cholesterol and promote healthy hair, nails and skin. Another way to get essential fat is to use <u>cold pressed oils such as rapeseed, extra virgin olive oil, walnut and sesame oil.</u>

Chapter Three
Eat the Rainbow

Antioxidants

Antioxidants come up frequently in discussions about good health and preventing diseases. These powerful substances, which mostly come from the fresh fruits and vegetables we eat, prohibit (and in some cases even prevent), the oxidation of other molecules in the body. The benefits of antioxidants are very important to good health, because if free radicals are left unchallenged, they can cause a wide range of illnesses and chronic diseases.

Antioxidants and Free Radicals

The human body naturally produces free radicals and the antioxidants to counteract their damaging effects. However, in most cases, free radicals far outnumber the naturally occurring antioxidants. In order to maintain the balance, and maximise the benefits of antioxidants a continual supply of external sources of antioxidants are necessary. Antioxidants benefit the body by neutralising and removing the free radicals from the bloodstream.

Different Antioxidants Benefit Different Parts of the Body

There are a wide range of antioxidants found in nature, and because they are so varied, different antioxidants provide benefits to different parts of the body. For example, beta-carotene (and other carotenoids) is very beneficial for healthy eyes, lycopene is beneficial for helping maintain prostate health; flavonoids are especially beneficial in maintaining a healthy heart; and proanthocyanins are beneficial for urinary tract health.

Antioxidants and Skin Health Benefits

When skin is exposed to high levels of ultraviolet light, photo-oxidative damage is induced by the formation of different types of reactive species of oxygen, including singlet oxygen, superoxide radicals, and peroxide radicals. These forms of reactive oxygen damage cellular lipids, proteins, and DNA, and they are considered to be the primary contributors to erythema (sunburn), premature aging of the skin, photo dermatoses, and skin cancers.

Antioxidants and Immune System Support

Singlet oxygen can compromise the immune system, because it has the ability to catalyze production of free radicals. Astaxanthin and Spirulina have been shown to enhance both the non-specific and specific immune system, and to protect cell membranes and cellular DNA from mutation. Astaxanthin is the single most powerful quencher of singlet oxygen, and is up to ten times stronger than other carotenoids (including beta-carotene), and up to 500 times stronger than alpha tocopherol (Vitamin E), while Spirulina has a variety of antioxidants and other substances that are beneficial in boosting immunity.

Additional Ways Antioxidants Help Benefit our Health

Increasing one's antioxidant intake is essential for optimum health, especially in today's polluted world. Because the body just can't keep up with antioxidant production, a good amount of these vitamins, minerals, phytochemicals, and enzymes must come from our daily diet. Boosting your antioxidant intake can help provide added protection for the body against heart problems, eye problems, memory problems, mood disorders and immune system problems.

Top Antioxidant – rich Fruit and Vegetables.

Blackberries, blueberries, broccoli, Brussel sprouts, Curly kale, garlic, plums, prunes, raisins, raspberries, red peppers, spinach and strawberries.

Plant Nutrients -

The more variety and colour you eat the more nutrients you will consume and the more benefit you will get from your diet.

According to a recent National Diet and Nutrition Survey many of our diets - adults and children - are lacking in vitamin A and D, selenium and zinc and many women are lacking calcium and iron.

Fruit and vegetables are considered so good for us that nutritionists suggest that the recommended government 5 a day should be our bare minimum. But the truth is that most people aren't even eating 5 a day. Fruit and vegetables provide a huge variety of vitamins, minerals and fibre and if you are missing out on eating them you will leave a big gap in the nutrients you consume.

The best way to get the most from your food is variety. Many people get stuck in a rut, eating the same food day in and day out with little or no variety. In order to stay healthy, the body needs over 40 different vitamins and minerals a day so sticking to the same foods will hugely reduce your intake.

Introducing new and different foods to your weekly shop will not only keep your food exciting but your body will reap the rewards.

Whilst some foods have significant health benefits it is important to remember that no one individual food can treat, prevent or cure health problems, the key is to eat all foods as part of a balanced diet.

Include fruit and vegetables from the five colour groups, red, orange, yellow, green and purple. Different coloured fruit and vegetables contain different nutrients, combining them is the best way to ensure you get all you need.

Many of the naturally occurring chemicals responsible for giving fruit and veg their bright colours actually help keep us healthy and free from disease. Fruit and vegetables contain hundreds of colourful phytochemicals that act as antioxidants.

Antioxidant-rich fruit and vegetables can help to protect against heart disease, cancer, and premature aging.

Red–

Many red foods contain high levels of vitamin C. They contain high levels of anthocyanins which are linked to being effective in fighting cancer, bacterial infections and neurological diseases.

Red fruit and vegetables to include in your diet

are raspberries, cranberries, strawberries, cherries, pomegranate, apples, rhubarb, red peppers, tomatoes and watermelon.

Orange

Orange fruit and vegetables are high in carotenoids, crucial for maintaining a good immune system and supporting cell repair and healthy vision.

Orange fruit and vegetables to include in your diet are Carrots, oranges, squashes, sweet potatoes, mangoes, peaches, nectarines, pumpkins, swede and peppers.

Yellow

Yellow fruit and vegetables contain large amounts of bioflavonoids, which fight infection and reduce inflammation.

Yellow fruit and vegetables to introduce into your diet – corn, pineapple, peppers and squashes.

Green

Green fruit and vegetables contain nutrients including lutein, lycopene, folic acid, zeaxanthin and glycosylates all of which are associated with helping to prevent cancer.

Green fruit and vegetables to include in your diet - asparagus, avocado, rocket, spinach, lettuce, watercress, cucumber, broccoli, Brussels sprouts, leafy cabbage, spring greens, beans, peas, sugar snap peas, mange tout, cress, courgette, peppers, spring onions, leeks, apples, grapes and kiwi fruit.

Purple/blue

Purple and blue fruit and vegetables are high in antioxidants which promote healthy blood and are believed to have antiaging properties.

Purple and blue fruit and vegetables to include in your diet are blackberries, blueberries, grapes, blackcurrants, plums, red cabbage, prunes, red onions, olives, purple sprouting broccoli, beetroot and aubergine.

Chapter Four

A Balanced Plate

Eat more than just the rainbow - As well as a variety of fruit, salad and vegetables we should also be eating beans, fish, nuts and seeds and good oils.

Beans –

Also known as pulses or legumes, pulses are packed with complete protein and contain almost no fat and are a good source of complex carbohydrates which are essential for good health.

Studies have linked that a higher consumption of beans results in a lower risk of heart disease and developing type 2 diabetes. It is now believed that a good intake of beans probably reduces the risk of stomach and prostate cancer.

Beans are low in fat and saturates and are packed with insoluble and soluble fibre, protein and a variety of minerals. Insoluble fibre helps keep our digestive system healthy whilst soluble fibre helps to control blood sugar levels and lowers cholesterol which means a lower risk of heart disease.

Beans provide potassium a nutrient that helps maintain fluid balance and helps to lower blood pressure. They also contain magnesium and phosphorus which strengthen bones. Many beans contain copper which gives us healthy skin and hair as well as a healthy immune system heart. Most beans provide manganese which is important for brain function and the metabolism of carbs and fat.

Beans are high in protein as well as good source of iron which makes them perfect for vegetarians and vegans. Because they contain both protein and fibre they keep us feeling fuller for longer. They help to slow down the absorption of sugar into the blood which means sugar levels stay even, this is not only good news for people trying to lose weight as it controls the appetite but also good news for people with type 2 diabetes who need to prevent dramatic rises in blood sugar.

Choose from - Aduki beans, black eyed beans, borlotti beans, chickpeas, fava beans, haricot beans, kidney beans, lentils, mung beans, soybeans and split peas.

Nuts –

There are many health benefits to eating nuts, they help lower your cholesterol, lower blood pressure and help you lose weight. The high fat content in nuts make them good for your heart because they are rich in polyunsaturated and monounsaturated fats which lower cholesterol.

Almonds – contain the most fibre, calcium and vitamin B2 which are good for healthy bones, skin, eyesight, red blood cells, nervous system and digestive system.

Brazil Nuts – have a very high selenium content, which is an antioxidant that is essential for a healthy immune system and protects against disease causing free radical damage.

Cashew Nuts – contain the most iron and make them a brilliant choice for vegetarians. Eat with vitamin C rich foods or a glass of orange juice to help the body absorb the iron more easily.

Peanuts – contain the least amount of calories and fat but the most amount of protein and B vitamins. Studies have also shown that people who ate a handful of peanuts twice a week significantly reduced their risk of bowel cancer.

Pistachios – has one of the lowest calories and fat content of other nuts and are the only nut to contain an antioxidant called lutein. Lutein is found in green vegetables and is good for healthy eyes.

Walnuts – are a great source of omega 3, walnuts contain alpha- linolenic acid which the body uses to make omega 3 fats that are found in oily fish such as salmon and mackerel.

Seeds –

Seeds are high in fats that are good for the heart as well as containing beneficial vitamins such as A, B, C, and E and nutrients such as iron, potassium, magnesium, phosphorus, copper, zinc and manganese. Just 30g of pumpkin seeds contain six times more iron then a small roasted chicken and 15% more than a small grilled rump steak, which makes them brilliant for vegetarians and vegans.

Sunflower seeds, flax seeds, alfalfa seeds, pumpkin seeds and sesame seeds are particularly beneficial. Seeds are so nutrient-dense that you don't have to eat a lot of them. Use them in cooking as garnishes or to flavour stews and casseroles, sprinkle them on soup, salads and roasted vegetables. Add them to cereals or smoothies or eat them as a snack.

Grains –

Grains are rich in nutrients and are basic energy foods. Almost all whole, unrefined grains can be beneficial to your health, generally the darker the colour the healthier it is.

Barley – pot barley is the wholegrain version. Barley is good for digestion. It is low in gluten.

Brown Rice – is beneficial for the nervous system and digestive system. It is the least allergenic of all grains. Basmati is perfect for people are overweight.

Buckwheat – is gluten free and rich in healthy minerals. A perfect choice for people who are sensitive to wheat. It is a good source of protein.

Millet – is high in iron, magnesium, potassium, the B vitamins and vitamin E. Millet helps to support the digestive system, improves nutrient uptake and is a great energy booster.

Quinoa – comes from South America. It contains all the essential amino acids and is therefore a complete protein but is easier to digest than meat protein and contains less fat.

Oats – contain more good fats then other grains. They are also a good source of vitamin B Complex which is good for the nervous system and for strengthening bones.

Spelt – like buckwheat is packed with minerals and protein. It is a good alternative for people who are sensitive to wheat, it helps stimulate the immune system and provides a good source of constant energy.

Fish –

Eating more fish is an important part of a healthy diet. Fish is a good source of protein. White fish and shellfish are low in fat and therefore low in calories. Studies have linked good intakes

of fish with a reduced risk of heart disease, depression, dementia and Alzheimer's disease. There is evidence that eating more fish may even reduce the risk of certain cancers.

<u>White Fish</u> – have a significant amount of B vitamins. White fish also contains iodine and selenium, nutrients that are essential for a healthy immune system.

Plaice – is particularly high in biotin which is needed for healthy hair and nails.

Sea Bream – is good for boosting vitamin B6 which is needed for making red blood cells.

Halibut – is one of the best sources of vitamin B3 which is essential for a healthy nervous system and releases energy from food.

Lemon sole and haddock – are good sources of iodine.

<u>Oil Rich Fish</u> – are packed with omega 3 fats which help prevent heart disease, heart attacks and strokes. Omega 3 fats are important for brain cell development particularly before babies are born and in the first few years of childhood.

Oily fish are also rich in vitamin D a nutrient that helps the body absorb calcium which keeps bones strong.

Sardines – not only contain calcium but also high levels of vitamin D.

Tuna (fresh not tinned) – contains high levels of selenium and iron which is an important nutrient for healthy blood.

Salmon – contains good amounts of omega 3 fats as well as being a particularly good source of vitamin E and vitamin B6.

Mackerel – contains one of the richest sources of omega 3 fats as well as iodine and vitamin D.

<u>Shellfish</u> – provide zinc which is essential for normal growth, enzyme function, wound healing, fertility and a healthy immune system.

Scallops – are particularly nutritious, they contain more selenium than either white fish or oily fish and tend to have more iron.

Muscles – are also a good source of iron.

Crab – is a good source of copper which is an important mineral for healthy hear and skin as well as a healthy immune and nervous system.

Prawns – have a higher cholesterol content then other fish but the cholesterol levels in prawns has little effect on blood cholesterol in the body and it is far more important to cut down on saturated fats.

Good Oils –

There are many different types of oils on the market, choosing the right one will bring nutritional value to your cooking.

On the whole oils contain less saturated fat then animal fats such as butter and lard. And more polyunsaturated and monounsaturated fats which can lower your cholesterol. Cooking oils which are liquid when kept at room temperature are mostly derived from plants, nuts and seeds. They all have a similar amount of calories, which is approx. 100kcal per 1 tbsp. but they differ in the type of fat they contain and their smoke point, which is the temperature at which they start to break down. When the smoke point is reached, the quality, flavour and nutritional benefits are affected. It is important to understand what oils are best for what type of use.

Ground Nut Oil – is made from peanuts and is wonderful for your heart. It is packed with plant sterols that can lower your risk of heart disease. Ground nut oil – as its name would suggest – has a slightly nutty but mild flavour and is very versatile. It has a high smoke point which makes it a good oil to use for grilling or frying.

Olive Oil – is rich in monounsaturated fats which boost good cholesterol and have a beneficial effect on your heart. Olive oil can be heated to higher temperatures which makes it perfect for grilling, baking, roasting or stirring through pastas.

Light Olive Oil – means that the oil is lighter in colour and flavour and it has a higher smoke point making it good for grilling and frying. The term "light" does not mean that it contains fewer calories or fat content.

Extra Virgin Olive Oil – is richer in antioxidants. It has a lower smoke point which means that it loses much of its nutritional benefits when heated. Use it for dressing and sauces that don't need to be cooked.

Rapeseed Oil – is a good all-rounder. Low in saturated fats and high in heart friendly monounsaturated fats rapeseed oil also contains omega 3 and vitamin E. This oil is great in salad dressings but also, because it has a high smoke point it is also perfect for frying, roasting and baking.

Sunflower Oil – is low in saturated fats, rich in polyunsaturated fat – omega 6, and vitamin E. It is a good all-purpose oil, its mild flavour makes it good for using in salads and dressings and its high smoke point means it is also good for frying, roasting and grilling.

Toasted Sesame Oil – is most associated with oriental dishes because of its rich, nutty flavour. It is a good sauce of oleic acid which is good for the heart. Its low smoke point means it is not good for cooking – unless you combine it with another oil, such as Olive or Sunflower oil. It is best used for its flavour in salad dressings or dips.

Chapter five

Rules for Healthy Living.

Cook from scratch

Take responsibility for what you are eating by knowing exactly what is in your food. Cooking from scratch doesn't have to be complicated or time consuming. look for quick, simple recipes, the fewer the ingredients the quicker the dish, and use good quality ingredients to maximise nutrition. Plan ahead and know what you are going to cook and adapt your menu to the time you have. The recipes in this plan will help you do just that.

Read the labels

Food labels are a reliable, accurate source of valuable nutritional information. Use the labels on the foods you buy to ensure that you are consuming what you think you are consuming. Ingredients are listed in descending order by weight and include any colour, additives, preservatives and, nutrients, fats or sugar that have been added to the product.

Whatever appears first on the list is the largest ingredient. Foods with high levels of sugar, salt or saturated fats at the top of the list should be avoided.

Know your Sugar

Sugar comes in many forms with many different names, but it is all the same and has the same effect on the body. Products with sugar listed at the top of its ingredients list is more than likely high in sugar. The following are all sugars – brown sugar, cane juice lactose, maltose, raw cane sugar, raw sugar, sucrose sugar, invert sugar, glucose, fructose, dextrose, corn syrup, corn sweetener.

Consider naturally sweet alternatives such as raw honey or maple syrup or add fruit such as apples, apricots and berries. Carrot or apple juice makes a great base for vegetable juices as they add sweetness.

Know Your Fats

Good fats or "essential fatty acids" as they are known come from nuts and seeds, fish and avocados, they are important for a healthy, balanced diet. These can also be added to your cooking by using them as oils such as sunflower and pumpkin seed oil, macadamia, coconut, walnut, hazelnut and olive oils are all beneficial fats that support nerve function, mental alertness, concentration and memory.

Bad fats or saturated / trans fats are known to raise levels of cholesterol and increase the risk of heart disease. These are found mainly in animal produce and dairy products they are in butter, lard, margarine, cooking fats, chocolate, biscuits, cakes, savory snacks and processed foods.

Read the label and avoid anything that says it contains "hydrogenated" or "partially hydrogenated oils"

Add colour

The more colour in your diet the more goodness you will consume. Each colour of fruit and vegetables contains different and important antioxidants. Antioxidants are part of a well- balanced, healthy diet, they will keep you well throughout the winter months by helping your immune system to kill harmful bacteria and infections and they will keep your skin and hair looking good and give you vitality. Vitamins A, C and E are all found in fresh fruit and vegetables and are all antioxidants.

Be prepared

Always make a meal plan and a shopping list before shopping. Consider the week ahead in advance. Think about foods that you love and how you can introduce more variety to them. Don't be afraid to find recipes and tweak them to suit your own tastes you may discover something wonderful.

Consider days that you might be home late or have more work to do than normal and make those evening meals simple and quick or even prepare them at the weekend, or when you have more time, and freeze them so that they are at hand when you need a quick meal. Making your own microwave meals doesn't need to be either complicated or time consuming – it just needs planning. Consider, omelets, stir fries or salads with fresh or tinned fish.

Stay Hydrated

Dehydration can, falsely, make you think that you are hungry. Your brain can confuse thirst with hunger. Before reaching for a biscuit or sweets make a conscious effort to have a glass of water and then decide whether you were hungry or thirsty. If you really are hungry consider what you are reaching for.

Healthy Snacking.

Snacking between meals is a good thing. As long as you make the right choices, healthy snacking keeps your blood sugars level and increases your energy. Snacking keeps your brain active meaning that you can concentrate and remain focused throughout the day and on into the evening.

If you enjoy your snacks, aim for fruit, plain or unsweetened Greek-style yogurt, celery sticks, carrots or nuts and seeds.

Not Just 5 a Day

We all know that 5 portions of fruit and vegetables a day is the recommended amount. Given the nutritional value in fruit and vegetables and the health benefits of them 5 portions should be your absolute minimum and whilst meal planning you should be looking at ways of increasing your consumption wherever you can.

Try adding fruit to your breakfast cereal or drinking a smoothie instead of a cup of tea for breakfast, be more adventurous with your salads, replace your lunchtime sandwich and crisps with a salad and add vegetables to your pasta sauces, stews and soups and before you know it you will have increased your intake of fruit and veg without even noticing.

Flavour Your Food with Herbs and Spices.

Spices have been found to inhibit the formation of prostaglandins – the hormones that trigger inflammatory reactions. Reduce your use of salt and increase your use of herbs and mild spices to flavour your food instead. Use - cloves, cinnamon, turmeric, rosemary, ginger, sage, and thyme all of which are known for their anti-inflammatory properties.

Scientists in India have found that curcumin, the primary active ingredient of turmeric, has anti – depressant qualities that were found to be at least as effective as certain medications in the treatment of depression – but without the negative side effects.

Refined V Unrefined

Always choose unrefined ingredients over refined ones.

Unrefined foods contain more natural nutrients because they have not been stripped of their vitamins and minerals in the refining process.

Fibre

People who eat a lot of refined foods and skip the fruit and vegetables are missing out on fibre. A lack of fibre in the diet leads to digestive problems and blood sugar imbalances. Fibre is the indigestible portion of grains, vegetables and fruit it is used by the body to improve intestinal function, helps to grow healthy bacteria in the gut and helps prevent disease by removing waste products and toxins from the body. Drop the white bread, pasta and rice and increase fruit, vegetables and whole grains wherever possible.

Eat at least 25 grams of fibre every day. A fibre-rich diet helps reduce inflammation by supplying the body with anti-inflammatory phytonutrients found in fruits, vegetables, and other whole foods. The best sources of fibre are whole grains, such as barley and oatmeal; vegetables such as peas, Brussel sprouts, parsnips and spinach, and fruit such as apples, bananas, oranges, strawberries and raspberries.

Chapter Six

Change Your Diet Change Your Life.

There are many tips and tricks that you can implement to help you get to sleep every night. One of the most underrated sleep practices that really goes far in improving quality sleep is making the right dietary choices.

Almost everybody is aware of the value that eating certain foods is instrumental in our daily lives. Eating the right foods gives us the energy we need to complete tasks, strengthen our immune system against diseases, improve cognitive functions, heal wounds, repair bones and tissues, help our children grow big strong, and basically everything else we need to live happy, healthy, productive lives. But too often healthy eating is rarely thought about when it comes to sleep. Your diet really can have amazing benefits in helping you get to sleep, and stay asleep.

The Best Foods for a Great Night's Sleep

There are four main vitamins and minerals that can be found in food that aid in promoting sleep: tryptophan, magnesium, calcium, and B6. Some of these substances help the body produce melatonin, the hormone that is responsible for regulating your circadian rhythm (sleep/wake patterns). When you're close to bedtime, melatonin production naturally increases to help you sleep. In the morning when you're ready to wake up, melatonin production tapers off to allow you to be awake and alert for the day.

Some foods are naturally packed with these essential vitamins and minerals, and eating certain foods at certain times can help you tip the scales towards a successful night of quality sleep. Most of these are available as over-the-counter supplements, but like with most supplements, it's better to get them from the foods you eat.

Tryptophan

Tryptophan is an amino acid that when ingested gets turned into the neurotransmitter serotonin and is then converted into the hormone melatonin. Here are some of the best foods loaded with tryptophan:

Dairy products (milk, low-fat yogurt, cheese)

Poultry (turkey, chicken)

Seafood (shrimp, salmon, halibut, tuna, sardines, cod)

Nuts and seeds (flax, sesame, pumpkin, sunflower, cashews, peanuts, almonds, walnuts)

Legumes (kidney beans, lima beans, black beans split peas, chickpeas)

Fruits (apples, bananas, peaches, avocado)

Vegetables (spinach, broccoli, turnip greens, asparagus, onions, seaweed)

Grains (wheat, rice, barley, corn, oats)

Magnesium

Magnesium is a powerful mineral that is instrumental in sleep and is a natural relaxant that helps deactivate adrenaline. A lack of magnesium can be directly linked to difficulty going and staying asleep. Magnesium is often referred to as *the* sleep mineral. Excellent sources of magnesium are:

Dark leafy greens (baby spinach, kale, collard greens)

Nuts and seeds (almonds, sunflower seeds, brazil nuts, cashews, pine nuts, flaxseed, pecans)

Wheat germ

Fish (salmon, halibut, tuna, mackerel)

Soybeans

Banana

Avocados

Low-fat yogurt

Calcium

Calcium is another mineral that helps the brain make melatonin. A lack of calcium can cause you to wake up in the middle of the night and have difficulty returning to sleep. Calcium rich diets have been shown to help patients with insomnia. Dairy products that contain both tryptophan and calcium are among the best sleep inducers. Sources of calcium include:

Dark leafy greens

Low-fat milk

Cheeses

Yogurt

Sardines

Fortified cereals

Soybeans

Fortified orange juice

Enriched breads and grains

Sugar snap peas

Okra

Broccoli

Vitamin B6

Vitamin B6 also helps convert tryptophan into melatonin. A deficiency in B6 has been linked with lowered serotonin levels and poor sleep. A deficiency in B6 is also linked to symptoms of depression and mood disorders which can lead to insomnia. Highest sources of B6 are:

Sunflower seeds

Pistachio nuts

Flaxseed

Fish (tuna, salmon, halibut)

Meat (chicken, tuna, lean pork, lean beef,)

Dried Prunes

Bananas

Avocado

Spinach

Melatonin

Many of the vitamins and minerals that are on this list are there because they help aid in the production of turning serotonin into melatonin. However, there are a few excellent sources of naturally occurring melatonin in foods:

Fruits and vegetables (tart cherries, corn, asparagus, tomatoes, pomegranate, olives, grapes, broccoli, cucumber)

Grains (rice, barley, rolled oats)

Nuts and Seeds (walnuts, peanuts, sunflower seeds, mustard seeds, flaxseed)

Drinks that will help you sleep

It's not just foods that are great for sleep. Many drinks contain essential vitamins and minerals that help aid with sleep. A few of the ones to try are:

Warm milk

Almond milk

Valerian tea

Chamomile tea

Tart cherry juice

Passion fruit tea

Peppermint tea

Chapter Seven

Eat More of the Right Foods

Tryptophan

Tryptophan's reputation is well-deserved: It makes you sleepy and helps keep you asleep for a good night's rest. It's also one of the essential amino acids that your body needs, yet can't make, so it must come from the proteins you eat. Poultry, fish and meats are among the best sources of tryptophan, but you'll also get it from the broccoli.

Because it's an amino acid, tryptophan helps make the proteins you need to build muscles and other tissues, but it's better known for other roles. Your body converts tryptophan into the neurotransmitter serotonin, which helps stabilize mood. Serotonin is then turned into the hormone melatonin. Melatonin regulates your sleep cycle by being produced and released based on the amount of light in your environment. Levels of melatonin are high after dark to help you sleep; the amount in your system drops during the day. The body also uses tryptophan to make niacin, which is essential for metabolism and making red blood cells.

The following foods are good sources of Tryptophan and when introduced into your daily diet can significantly reduce problems with insomnia.

Almonds and Almond Milk

A great muscle-relaxing magnesium source comes from nuts. Cashews and peanuts are good, but almonds are great. Almonds are also high in calcium. The combination of magnesium and calcium work together to calm the body and relax muscles. Calcium plays its role by helping the brain convert the amino acid tryptophan into sleep-inducing melatonin. This also explains why dairy products which contain both tryptophan and calcium, are one of the top sleep-inducing foods.

Eat more nuts: - Eat a handful of mixed nuts as a snack, sprinkle chopped nuts onto yoghurt, cereal and salad, add them to your morning smoothie. Nut butters can be eaten with dried fruit, added to baking or spread on toast, try nut milks as an alternative to cow milk.

Avocado

Avocados contain good fats which balance blood sugar, plus a ton of fibre. They also have a lot of magnesium which is a wonderful nutrient for relaxation and helping aid natural sleep.

Eat more avocados: - Mash them on toast, add them to salads, blitz them in pesto and add them to pasta.

Bananas

Bananas are an excellent source of both potassium and magnesium, bananas can put your body into a sleepy state by helping with muscle relaxation. Magnesium has a positive effect on the quality of sleep in older adults with insomnia by extending the time they spent sleeping in bed (rather than just lying there) and making it easier to wake up. Bananas also contain tryptophan, the precursor to calming and sleep-regulating hormones serotonin and melatonin.

Eat more bananas: - add them to your cereal, blend them in smoothies add them to yoghurt, milk or fruit salad. Split the skins, wrap them in tin foil and add them to the barbeque – for a little more luxury pour a little brandy into the tin foil before cooking and once cooked serve with cream or ice cream.

Broccoli

One cup of chopped, raw broccoli contains 30 milligrams of tryptophan. Along with dairy products and leafy greens, broccoli is a great source of calcium. Research has shown that a calcium deficiency can cause sleep disturbances. Vitamin A deficiencies can also cause sleep problems, especially in older adults and those suffering from Parkinson's disease, Alzheimer's disease, schizophrenia and depression.

Eat more broccoli: - steam it on the side with a sprinkling of mixed seeds, add it to soups, quiches and stir fries.

Chamomile

Drinking a cup of chamomile tea just before bed will help you sleep. According to researchers, drinking the tea is associated with an increase of glycine, a chemical that relaxes nerves and muscles and acts as a mild sedative.

Drink more Chamomile Tea: - Drink a cup of soothing chamomile tea in the evening when you want to unwind. Chamomile is in flower in June, make the most of it and use it fresh in teas, salads and fritters.

Cheeses

Eating a small snack before bed can stop you waking feeling hungry in the night. Opt for a slice of whole grain bread with a little cottage cheese. Cottage cheese is rich in casein protein which is a slow releasing milk protein that will keep hunger at bay through the night—it also contains the amino acid tryptophan. Mix it with humous for an added tryptophan boost, or with guacamole for some muscle-relaxing magnesium.

Eat more Cheese: - Low fat cheese such as cottage cheese or cream cheese eaten with whole grain bread makes a great light snack before bed.

Cherries

Studies have shown that people who drank just one ounce of tart cherry juice a day reported that they slept longer and more soundly than those who didn't. Cherries act as a natural sleep aid due to their melatonin content, a naturally produced hormone that signals to our bodies that it's time for bed.

Eat more Cherries: - Add fresh cherries to fruit salads, an evening bowl of whole grain cereal or enjoy a glass of juice.

Dairy Products

Drinking a glass of warm milk before bed could help you fall asleep more quickly. Milk is an excellent source of magnesium, which, has been found to be associated with deeper, less-interrupted sleep. Milk and other dairy foods, such as cheese and yogurt, are also high in calcium, which helps the brain make melatonin, a sleep-inducing hormone.

Eat more Dairy: - low fat cheese, such as cream cheese or cottage cheese make excellent evening snacks as do warm milky drinks or milk and whole grain cereal.

Eggs

Eggs are high in vitamin A, but make sure you eat the whole egg, as the yolk contains 100 percent of the vitamin A found in an egg.

Eat more eggs: - have them poached, boiled, omelet or scrambled, eat them for breakfast, in your packed lunch or in salads.

Fortified Cereals

A low-sugar cereal paired with skim milk is a perfect bedtime snack. Milk contains the amino acid tryptophan, which converts to the hormone serotonin, a sleep-inducing agent.

Honey

Just one teaspoon of honey is enough to stimulate the release of melatonin in the brain and shut off orexin (which keeps us alert), thus helping you to wind down.

Eat more Honey: - Add a spoon full of honey to a cup of herbal tea before bed, drizzle it on cereal or yoghurt for a light evening snack.

kiwi

Studies show that people who consumed two kiwifruits 1 hour before bedtime nightly for 4 weeks fell asleep 35 percent faster than those who didn't eat them. Besides being rich in antioxidants, carotenoids, and vitamins C and E, it also contains the hormone, serotonin. Kiwi is also rich in folate, and insomnia is one of the health issues that is a symptom of folate deficiency.

Eat more Kiwi: - Add them to salads and fruit salads, yoghurts, smoothies and cereals or simply peeled and sliced.

Leafy Greens

Green leafy vegetables like kale are loaded with calcium,

which helps the brain use tryptophan to manufacture melatonin. Spinach and mustard greens are other good options.

A deficiency in folic acid has been associated with insomnia, so eating foods high in folate, such as lentils, may improve sleep. Lentils are best enjoyed in soups or cold salads. Cauliflower, beets, parsley and asparagus are also good sources of folate. Green leafy vegetables, such as spinach, kale, romaine lettuce and collard greens, are also high in folate, as well as calcium and magnesium, two other power nutrients for sleep. A diet high in folate can also help combat chronic fatigue syndrome.

Eat more Greens: - Steam them, add them to soups and stews, smoothies and salads.

Legumes

Beans and other legumes are packed with vitamin B s, such as B6, B12, and folic acid—all of which help you to regulate your sleep/ wake cycles and boost your natural levels of serotonin, a feel-good, relaxing hormone.

Eat more beans: - Make shepherd's pie or lasagna with beans or lentils instead of mince, add them cold to salads, put them in stews and soups. Make pates, humous and pesto sauce with them.

Lemon Balm Tea

A relaxing tea is lemon balm. Studies have found that lemon balm serves as a natural sedative, and researchers reported that they observed reduced levels of sleep disorders among people who regularly drank a cup of Lemon Balm Tea before bed.

Drink more Lemon Balm Tea: - Hot in the winter or chilled in the summer it's a great relaxant before bed.

Low fat Yoghurt

Combine low-fat Greek yogurt, honey, banana and a handful of oats. Yogurt, oats and bananas all contain tryptophan, and the carbs from the banana will help the tryptophan-rich foods get absorbed by the brain.

Eat more live bio yoghurt: - eat it for breakfast with fruit and a sprinkling of chopped nuts or mixed seeds. Add it to sauces or have it on the side of salads or curries.

Nuts/ Seeds

Nuts are a good source of tryptophan, a sleep-enhancing amino acid that helps make serotonin and melatonin, the "body clock" hormone that sets your sleep-wake cycles.

Nuts such as pecans, walnuts and almonds, and seeds such as pumpkin, sunflower, sesame and flax, also contain magnesium. In addition, those same nuts contain tryptophan, which can improve depression and promote relaxation.

Eat more nuts: - Eat a handful of mixed nuts as a snack, sprinkle chopped nuts onto yoghurt, cereal and salad, add them to your morning smoothie. Nut butters can be eaten with dried fruit, added to baking or spread on toast, try nut milks as an alternative to cow milk.

Passion Flower Tea

Many herbal teas offer sedative effects through their flavones, flavonoids, and resins. Passionflower tea is known to have anti-anxiety benefits and is a mild sedative, helping you calm nervousness so you can sleep at night.

Drink more Passion Flower Tea: - With a spoon of honey drink a cup of passion flower tea before bed for a relaxing night's sleep.

Peas

Peas' help regulate your brain activity during sleep. They also help you produce melatonin, a hormone in your brain that controls your daily sleep/ wake cycle.

Eat more Peas: - Add fresh peas to salads and pastas, add cooked peas to stews and soups, blitz them into dips, spreads and sauces

Peppermint Tea

Drinking peppermint tea before bed has been proven to give you a more restful sleep it helps the relaxation of the muscles which leads to a more restful sleep.

Drink more Peppermint Tea: - Hot in the winter or chilled in the summer, a cup of peppermint tea before bed will ensure a restful sleep.

Seafood

A good source of tryptophan are crustaceans like shrimp or lobster as well as oily fish which may bring on a more restful sleep.

Eat more fish: - Mackerel, salmon, sardines and tuna are the most obvious choices. Try to eat 2 / 3 servings a week. Eat fish poached, baked or grilled, cook them on the barbeque, make fish pie or fish pate, flake them into salad.

Spinach

Not only is spinach a source of tryptophan, the green is an excellent source of folate, magnesium, and vitamins B6 and C, which are all key co-factors in synthesizing serotonin, and subsequently, melatonin. Spinach also contains glutamine, an amino acid which stimulates the body to get rid of the cellular toxins that lead to sleeplessness. Cooking spinach breaks down the glutamine as well as vitamins C and B.so its best eaten raw.

Eat more spinach: - Eat it fresh in salad, or cooked as a vegetable. Make pesto with it, put it in an omelett, add it to potatoes for a pie filling or blend it in your morning smoothie.

Valerian Tea

Valerian is an herb that's long been valued as a mild sedative. Studies have shown that 30% of people who drank Valerian Tea before bed reported an improvement in the quality of their sleep.

Drink more Valerian Tea: - With a spoon of honey, a cup of valerian tea just before bed will ensure a restful night.

Warm Milk

Drinking a glass of warm milk will help you fall asleep. Milk contains tryptophan which when released into the brain produces serotonin.

Drink more Warm Milk: - try steeping a bag of chamomile tea into warm milk with a spoonful of honey for a bedtime treat or poured over a small bowl of whole grain cereal which will not only help you sleep more soundly it will also keep hunger away through the night.

Whole Grains

The "whole" part is important. Whole grains include the germ of the grain, which is removed during the refining of whole wheat grains into white flour. This germ includes important B vitamins such as folate and vitamin B6—both important micronutrients required for proper absorption of tryptophan—as well as magnesium to loosen your muscles.

People who are deficient in magnesium often experience long-term sleep deprivation. You can combat a lack of magnesium in your diet with whole-grain foods such as quinoa, barley, bulgur, whole-grain breads and pastas, whole oats and brown rice.

Eat more whole grains: - Look for whole grain alternatives to the normal white bread, pasta and rice. Eat more porridge, muesli and wholegrain cereals. Add cooked grains to salads, stews and soups.

Chapter Eight

Foods to Avoid

Break Bad Food Habits

Just as there are foods and drinks that help promote sleep, there are also foods to avoid that can rob you of sleep. Many of the foods to avoid on this list are healthy for you to eat, but just not recommended to eat before bed because they can interfere with sleep.

Alcohol.

Alcohol does not help promote sleep. While it can make you drowsy and more likely to fall asleep faster, it often disrupts sleep and can deter you from entering the deeper, much needed phases of the sleep cycles.

Caffeine.

If you have problems with sleeping it's not recommended that you drink caffeine in the early evening (and especially near bedtime), as it can interfere with sleep by keeping your mind overactive. Foods with dark chocolate are also high in caffeine and should be avoided late in the day.

Saturated Fat

High levels of fat in your diet have been linked to poor, fragmented sleep. Fat triggers the digestive processes and causes a build up of stomach acids, which can cause discomfort. A high fat diet also interferes with the production of orexin, one of the neurotransmitters that helps regulate your sleep/wake cycle along with melatonin.

Spicy foods.

While spicy foods are known to have many noted health benefits, eating spicy foods too close to bedtime can interfere with sleep. Spicy foods are known to cause heartburn, indigestion, and acid reflux. Heartburn can be made worse while lying down as it allows the acids to creep up into the oesophagus and burn the sensitive lining.

Foods high in protein

can also disrupt sleep when eaten too close to bedtime. Protein is tougher for the digestive system to break down. Eating protein rich meals near bedtime causes the body to spend more time working on digestion rather than focusing on sleeping.

Foods containing water

such as watermelon and celery are natural diuretics which help push water through your system. Eating these types of foods and drinking anything too close to bedtime can cause you to lose sleep from middle of the night bathroom trips.

Heavy meals before bedtime.

As with most things in life, moderation is the key. Even

eating too much of the recommended foods before bed can cause you to lose sleep because your body is focused on digestion. If you find yourself hungry before bed, a light snack is recommended. The best light snacks are those that contain tryptophan and calcium such as a bowl of cereal, cheese and crackers, or peanut butter on toast.

While the author has made every effort to ensure that the information contained in this book is as accurate and up to date as possible, it is advisory only and should not be used as an alternative to seeking specialist medical advice. The author cannot be held responsible for actions that may be taken by the reader as a result of reliance on the information contained in this book, which are taken entirely at the readers own risk.